What's the Next Step?

What's the Next Step?

ROBERT FRITZ

What's the Next Step?
My journey with cancer as a caregiver and then as a caretaker

iUniverse books may be ordered through booksellers or by contacting:

iUniverse
1663 Liberty Drive
Bloomington, IN 47403
www.iuniverse.com
1-800-Authors (1-800-288-4677)

ISBN: 978-1-4502-9631-1 (pbk)
ISBN: 978-1-4502-9630-4 (cloth)
ISBN: 978-1-4502-9632-8 (ebk)

Printed in the United States of America

iUniverse rev. date: 1/27/2011

This book is dedicated to my wife, Li Vellinga.

The words *my best friend* make a poor crown for her

lovely head, but they're the best I have.

She always speaks of "*we* have an appointment" and

"what are *our* blood tests showing."

I will love her always.

Contents

Preface

Adjusting to a life-threatening illness is akin to finding yourself dropped at the base of Mt. Everest and being told to start climbing. It is a difficult task at best, but a guide can show you the tools and techniques to make the journey much easier. And thus you can get some time to enjoy the view, now and then.

There is a view worth seeing, too, like in the community where I live on the banks of Rock Creek. You can take in a panorama of friends you never guessed you had; relish in the warmth in the genuine caring of a spouse; feel the lightness that comes from dropping the rocks of anger from your backpack; feel a freedom from worry about the unknown; and know the joy that comes from doing that thing that you always wanted to do. You can live, perhaps for the first time.

This little book is based on my diary as I went from being just another retired Silicon Valley engineer thinking about when to apply for Social Security to, in the space of a week, wondering if I would live to see that day.

The story, though, does not start with me. I lost my previous wife, Mary Jane, after she battled breast cancer for thirteen years. She gave me the gift of a graceful passing. In doing so I have discovered some real, practical tools that I would like to pass on.

Although there is solace to be found in religion, science, and studying the writings of innumerable philosophers, they take a leap of faith or too long to study. Here, I ask you only to use what you already know.

> IF YOU'RE RELIGIOUS, REJOICE;
> THERE'S A BETTER WORLD AWAITING YOU.

And so you will find pages with blank lines, not because I had nothing else to say, it is for you to make comments as you read, discuss your own experience, or simply to remember the journey of someone you love. Making a graceful climb can be done. But it requires a conscious effort.

Bob Fritz

Sierra Foothills

The photograph on the cover by Victor Valdez
shows Rock Creek taken from a bridge above on Rock Creek Road
north of Placerville, CA. Book design: Jamie K. Hartshorn

> MOST PEOPLE ARE ABOUT AS HAPPY AS THEY
> MAKE UP THEIR MINDS TO BE.
> — ABRAHAM LINCOLN

ABE'S COMMENTS SOUND RATHER FACETIOUS. BUT CONSIDER THIS: THIS WAS A MAN LIVING IN THE MIDDLE OF A CIVIL WAR, WHO WAS AT THE TIME KNOWN TO BE A REAL JOKE TELLER. HE WAS ONCE STOPPED ON THE STREET BY A LITTLE OLD LADY AND ASKED, "MR. LINCOLN, IN THESE TIMES WHY ARE YOU ALWAYS TELLING JOKES?" HE REPLIED, "WELL MA'M, IF I DON'T KEEP LAUGHING, SURELY I'LL CRY."

The Journey Begins

For me the journey started in 1984 when Mary Jane and I were still dating and she informed me that she had breast cancer. We were confronted with statements of condolence that were usually more of a burden than a help.

We got married anyway, figuring that if the number of days were to be cut short we would best not waste them.

Now that I have stepped out of the doctor's tent at base-camp, so to speak, and started climbing my own mountain, the statements have returned. But having seen this situation from both sides I have gained a perspective that was, at first, expressed as anger at these people. More recently it has become one of an understanding with occasional forgiving. Those two characteristics are not necessarily linked; one can understand say, a criminal act without forgiving it. But the sequence must be in that order if you are to find peace within.

My goal here is to help both the consoler and the patient to that understanding. If you recognize yourself in these descriptions, and your feelings become a bit bruised, I apologize. My goal is not to punish, but to help. If your own journey has added some thoughts, please pass them on to:

bob@bobfritz.com or go onto my blog at

http://whatsthenextstep-swansborobob.blogspot.com/

LIFE IS A SPIRAL. YOU GO FULL CIRCLE MANY TIMES.
THE ROTATIONS USE THE TIME TO TAKE YOU TO A NEW PLACE
WHERE YOU CAN STILL SEE, BUT NOT REPEAT THE LESSONS.

Why are we so clumsy when death is near?

If you live to the typical age of about seventy years, death of someone you know will happen, perhaps several times. Oddly, we don't seem to get much better in our response.

We live in an age that insulates us from death. In centuries past, several generations lived under the same roof and we, as children, were trained to see and accept death. In our insulated single-family homes we can no longer take advantage of the lessons taught by elders, who had, in turn, learned from their elders.

My case is an example of a reinvent-the-wheel learning path. This writing started as anger at well-intentioned, but not too effective, attempts at cheering me up. Later, it became more of a diary. Now, I'm finding it helpful as I try to come to grips with the nature of this destruction of my body. Even still, I have to come back to what I have advised, reminding myself to stay on-track. It is not so easy.

The Tool Box

There are three keys to open this tool box. First, realize that regardless of any natural skills or prior training, all of us climb our own mountain. But it is largely a matter of choice as to what we make of the journey.

Second, realize that those who make a graceful ascent are human, just like us. They simply are using some tools; not some innate talent.

QUIT BUYING INTO THE IDEA THAT YOU HAVE TO SUBJECT

YOURSELF TO THE NEGATIVE INPUT.

Third, understand that you have the same tools right at hand. You need only to look and pick them up. But to use these tools, you must be in charge. You, not the feelings of panic, must be the boss.

TIME IS TOO SHORT.

DON'T WASTE TOO MUCH OF IT IN TEARS OR ANGER.

Tool #1 – Emotional Control

Keep your emotions in check. This will be difficult, but a moment of thought will reveal that in climbing the mountain, there are an infinite number of ways to make it difficult, but only a few ways to make it easier. It is unlikely that allowing emotion to be your guide will find that best path.

This is not ignoring the problem; it is not likely that it will just blow away on the breeze, so don't pretend that it will.

Emotions do have their place. The love of my friends is fabulous; the joy I feel in a just-do-it attitude is a heart-lightener; learning the meaning of "don't sweat the small stuff" is an emotionally refreshing bath. Keeping your emotions under control also has the benefit of allowing people to come to you, not be scared off. Emotion is not the guide; it is the pay-off when you find a beautiful view on the climb.

Emotional control is the single most important tool and will be repeated because without a grip on this, all else becomes difficult, if not outright impossible. When making decisions or feeling overwhelmed, you can ask yourself:

"Who's in charge? My emotions or intellect?"

This is a useful mantra beyond the realm of the malady that caused you buy this book, but it is a vital step to making this climb easier.

NOW IS THE TIME TO PLANT FLOWERS, NOT DIG A GRAVE.

Tool #2 – Know That You Are Not Alone

The second tool is an outgrowth of the first. Although everyone has, or will, climb their own mountain, the logical observation is that others have done this well. Know that you can too.

To use this tool you must first understand that it can be a graceful ascent. And by so doing you give yourself and your loved ones a gift that money cannot buy.

Let's hike over those fields of loose rocks that are at the beginning of the climb. And, like crossing a creek, the toughest part can be getting into the rhythm of the way.

Know that your friends want to help, and recognize that you will be hard pressed to hide the situation from your coworkers. Denial is an enemy that you can defeat! I have found that by being open about my illness, acquaintances have become friends and friends have become family. I sincerely mean this.

Last month thirty-eight people, several dogs, eight golf carts and a go-kart showed up at my workshop for a surprise birthday party on my behalf knowing that it would be fun; that we could talk about anything.

Denial of reality will only make the climb painful. Discuss it with your spouse or best friend. When someone asks how you feel, invite them for a hug to find out. Or just say "working on it" and drop it. We will get into the snappy retorts later.

> GIVE EVERY MAN THY EAR, FEW THY COUNSEL.
>
> — WILLIAM SHAKESPEARE
>
> LISTEN MORE THAN TALK.

Tool #3 – Finding the Internal Controls

The Kübler-Ross model, commonly known as the five stages of grief, was first introduced by Dr. Elisabeth Kübler-Ross in her 1969 book, *On Death and Dying*. It describes, in five discrete stages, a process by which people deal with grief and tragedy, especially when diagnosed with a terminal illness or catastrophic loss.

The Five Stages of Grief

1. **Denial** — "This can't be happening, not to me!"

2. **Anger** — "Why me? It's not fair!"

3. **Bargaining** — "I'll do anything for a few more years."

4. **Depression** — "I'm going to die! What's the point?"

5. **Acceptance** — "It's going to be okay. I may as well prepare for it."

What's not included is that those people who go through these stages are doing so as victims of the situation; they've not taken control of it. Again, we need to rely on logical thought, not emotion if we are to move over these areas of loose rock.

For me as a cancer caretaker, one essential tool has been the constant use of a mantra I coined:

"What's the next step?"

Keeping that at the forefront can help the patient literally glide through those stages of grief without falling off the edge into a canyon of despair.

Here is a situation that you have probably already had: Many are the times I have taken a one-week vacation and, upon arrival, the first thought is "Six days to go!" And on day two I say the same thing minus one day. Pretty soon I'm focusing on the end instead of the next step, and the vacation is a bust.

"Stop it!" I have to say to myself. What's going on this afternoon or tomorrow? That is, what's the next step?

The next step is not some distant action; it is what you will do in the next day or even hour. It could be as mundane as to clean up the workshop or kitchen. But it should not be to have a shot of whiskey or drown in anxiety. The purpose of this mantra is to get you thinking of a positive action. While a good scotch is, well, good, it is an escape. And cleaning up the workshop might be drudgery, but it is to accomplish something; something that works toward a future, which is there.

Initially I was told I had three months to live. Had I escaped into a bottle and had only three months, they would not have been much to be remembered by. As I write this, fifteen months have passed. Those three months were not pleasant, but I can look back and see how much I was and am loved. And I can be proud that I did not create a larger problem for those I love.

YOU'LL DO IT IMPERFECTLY. SO WILL THOSE YOU LOVE.
GIVE YOURSELF PERMISSION TO BE KIND TO YOURSELF
AND TO THEM.

Tool #4 – Enlightened Self-Interest

The 18th century French philosopher Voltaire developed a concept he called "Enlightened Self-Interest" after he observed that no one does anything without receiving something in return.

If I insist on always picking up the check at dinner, my guests get paid with a dinner and I get paid by their thank you's.

An enlightened approach though, strives for a more equitable balance. The too-generous person at dinner should let the other person pick up the check once in awhile.

So it is with the patient and the caregiver/visitor. I, as the patient, try to make it easy on those who say "Is there anything I can do?" by giving them something to do. I receive their gift, even if it is as simple as asking them to open a window; they get paid by knowing that they were of help, if only in a small way.

There's one more way in which you, the patient, can even help the person that says something callous or even painful. Gently but firmly point out that what they said wasn't helpful and then suggest that it would have been better had they simply asked, "What's the next step?" You've taken charge of the situation and you've helped them. You both get paid.

> TO EASE ANOTHER'S HEARTACHE IS TO FORGET ONE'S OWN.
> — ABRAHAM LINCOLN

Tool #5 – Just the Facts

First off, work hard at not speculating, guessing, or indulging in hope based on an internet search. This seems an obvious tool, but it is frequently left to rust.

Wonderful tool that the internet is, it can be your worst enemy too. The oft-repeated story of someone taking an ache or pain to full-blown hypochondria is real; researching an illness can scare you silly.

On the other side of the issue, researchers at Maastricht University in the Netherlands did a study which showed that a fear of the unknown was far more depressing than knowing the truth.

But what's the truth?

Start by trusting your doctor, but not blindly so; learn the basic jargon, but concentrate your efforts on the next step. We will get into the dreaded second-opinion later.

In my case, I have a Glioblastoma multiforme, stage 4 cancer. In simple terms, or so the first physician told me, it means I have a brain cancer that even with treatment, will take my life in about a year. But, here I am fifteen months later working on this project.

So don't fixate on a number; I have gotten projections ranging from three months to two years, had discussions with people who've been under treatment for twenty years and found an internet source promising a cure. What answer would you like?

> YOU DON'T EVER WANT A CRISIS TO GO TO WASTE;
> IT'S AN OPPORTUNITY TO DO IMPORTANT THINGS THAT YOU
> WOULD OTHERWISE AVOID.
> — RAHM EMANUEL

It all started for me with a seizure as I sat at my desk just as I am now. One second I was fiddling around with a birthday gift, the next second I was trying to focus on the faces of several emergency medical technicians who were attempting to put an oxygen mask on me with limited success because I kept battling it away.

The subsequent EEG measuring brain-wave activity didn't look right, so a CT scan was done and it also showed something suspicious. After about eight hours my wife drove me home and we prepared to go to a larger facility that could put some resolution to the initial tests.

We live in small community where an ambulance with red lights flashing in front of the house was an immediate cause for discussion throughout the area. Everyone quickly knew that something was amiss.

After the thirteen years of insensitive questions regarding my previous wife's situation I did not joyfully anticipate their questions, especially when I knew so little about the situation.

> SORROW SHARED IS HALVED.
>
> JOY SHARED IS DOUBLED.

Tool #6 – Fencing with the Physician

Are you a physician? Are you trained in this specialty? If not, you don't have a prayer of understanding the jargon especially at the pace it's going to come at you.

But you can distill it with a couple of tools.

First, let the doctor start, but don't be afraid to interrupt him with questions. "Excuse me, what's a hematoma?" or any other term you don't understand. It is your body he is explaining and it's your money (even via insurance) so get an explanation.

Second, ask how the procedure is performed. In my case it was brain surgery so, as a retired mechanical engineer, I wanted to see the design of the tools used to cut the bone, know if I'll have a large plate to replace the bone or would they put the bone back, etc. I found that knowing how it is done was a great emotional salve. That may well have been too scary for some, but for me it was a distraction and, hence, helpful.

Start asking these questions at the first meeting. If the doctor is annoyed by this, get a different doctor.

Tool #7 – Straight Answers That Are Not

Trusting your doctor is not the same as blindly trusting your doctor. The first doctor told me that patients in my situation have a "median of three months to live". After the first surgeon removed the tumor I was told that I had a median of twelve months. The tumor returned, was removed and that surgeon extended my median to two years.

Three doctors giving three numbers that vary by that much can induce more panic than understanding. Fortunately the number was going the right way. The confusion is easily smoothed by the knowledge that each doctor had more information than the previous one. The point here is that you should not fixate on a single opinion or number.

Understanding is taken to the next level by looking at the word "median", the definition of which is that half the patients lived longer than that number, and half lived less.

My favorite book in college? *How to Lie With Statistics* by Darrell Huff.

But there's a bit more to it. Take that last value of two years; it could mean half of them survived twenty three months and everyone was gone by month twenty five. Or it could be that patients passed away in equal numbers every month. The point here is that without knowing the shape of the curve, all I really know is that the chances of being around beyond that two-year mark are low and getting lower.

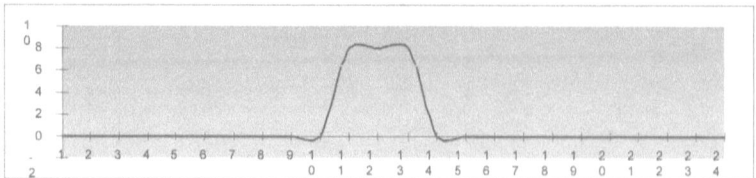

In the scenario above no one died prior to the tenth month and every-one was gone by the fourteenth month. But the median is still twelve months. If this were your graph, the message is not to worry until month ten and have a party at month fifteen, if you make it this far. Somebody has to make it to the extreme end.

> ## THE SINGLE MOST IMPORTANT QUESTION TO KEEP ASKING YOURSELF: WHO'S IN CHARGE? YOUR EMOTIONS OR YOUR INTELLECT?

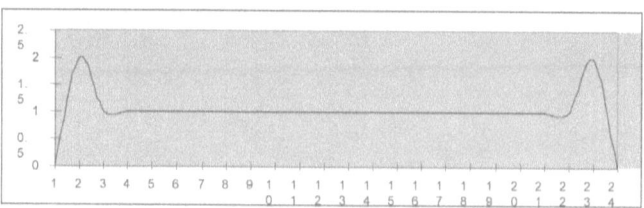

Here is the same twelve-month median, but now two people passed away in months two and twenty-three, and one per month in between.

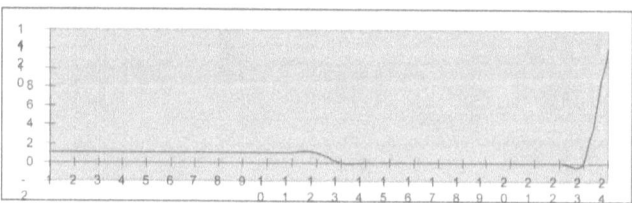

And here, one person passes every month for the first year, then the remainder left us in the twenty-fourth month. Clearly, if you make it through the first year, you've got a free ticket for the next year but not much longer.

Now, keep in mind that none of the above graphs are likely to be yours; in fact, mine probably bears no resemblance to them. But all three have the same median.

If you're put off by graphs or this seems a bit too technical to grasp, let me put it this way: you've got your left foot in a bucket filled with ice and your right foot in painfully hot water. The median is half way between those values so you must be comfortable. No?

DON'T LET SPECULATION STAMPEDE YOU.
JUST FOCUS ON THE NEXT STEP.

Truth be told, you need to know that other, more familiar statistical measure "Mean" (add the values and divide by the number of values), along with the standard deviation. But even if you did have that information and you understood it, you're still short of having the whole story for several more reasons.

My curve? I have referred to it several times but truth be known, I have no idea what it looks like. There are too many variables to be able to assign an individual to a given curve. This was the main reason this latest physician moved me out to two years saying "You're a youngish sixty-one."

A few months later all the good words evaporated when I asked if I should consider a change in diet.

"No, eat whatever you want" sounded at first like permission to party. I was tempted to let emotion take charge and have a ball, but something just didn't sit right. Keeping intellect in charge brought me around to the problem. The underlying message was that the situation is hopeless, just go for anything you want. In other words, eat drink and be merry, for tomorrow you die.

Again, a professional with experience in this field had spoken one thought and said another. His concern was that I would become focused on an extreme diet fed by false hopes, forgetting to enjoy what time I have. If you do even a quick look at the internet you'll find several books promising a miraculous cure if you'll eat bulgur (a sort of rice), no sugar, or any one of a number of combinations. To paraphrase Arlo Guthrie, "You can get any opinion you want, at the Internet restaurant."

IF IT SOUNDS TOO GOOD TO BE TRUE,

IT PROBABLY IS.

The doctor could have avoided this message if he'd simply explained that a lot of research had been done on diet, but no clear connection had been found between cancer remission and what you eat. He then should have spoken about the health benefits of simply eating right. That would have given the same message of avoiding useless pursuits for however much time I have while avoiding the negative implications. Remember to have thought, not emotion, in charge.

DON'T FORGET THAT YOU HAVE A GIFT.
YOU HAVE BEEN REMINDED TO TELL THE ONES YOU LOVE HOW
YOU FEEL, AND TO DO IT NOW. BUT IF YOU HAVE LIMITED TIME IT
MAKES LITTLE SENSE TO WASTE IT ON ANGER AND CREATING NEW
RESENTMENTS OR NURTURING OLD ONES.

What it all means

I have to stress that this is not to give you either unsubstantiated hope or imply deception on the part of the doctors; but then, you don't want to take that median as a fixed, not-to-exceed number either. Substitute "more-or-less" for "median" and you'll have a better sense of it.

A good example of this was my previous wife, MJ. She was told that she had "three to five years". That gives a much better, though not perfect, feel to the situation. Our response for the next thirteen years was to live as if we had only three years left. We took scuba lessons and went to Fiji and the Great Barrier Reef, toured England and found time to see the leaves turn in a New England Fall.

So, if your doctor tells you a median, respond with "What's the range for 75% of the patients?" And then don't fixate on that value either; as you've guessed, MJ was especially responsive to treatment and lived for thirteen years; somebody has to be out at the end of the curve.

My take on this time-remaining aspect has undergone some radical trans-formations since that first "well-informed" physician told me that I had three months to live. As you can imagine, that was a devastating thing to hear, and it got worse as he continued to speak.

In short, I have quit digging my grave and started planning in a some-what more positive fashion.

Tool #8 – The Second Opinion

Second opinions may be in agreement with the first opinion, or not. You could go to a third doctor and decide by voting, but chances are good you'll simply remain confused. Unless you're an MD and a specialist in the field, how do you evaluate any of them?

Listen to the doctor, as well, as the words. In my case, the first physician sounded almost terrified as he scared both my wife and me so this was not someone with whom we felt at ease.

The second physician spoke in enthusiastic terms of how he wanted to work with us, but was slow in returning phone calls. Scratch him from the list. Be careful to not obsess on their behavior, just drop 'em and move on. Your time is all that counts so don't spend it on dead-end pursuits.

Doctor three/surgeon#1 was young, confident, and defeatist in his telling us that he wouldn't do a second operation. If the chemo and radiation following the surgery didn't take care of the problem, his advice was to give up and enjoy what time was remaining.

This had an element of good advice in that we should avoid the charlatans and go on living. But it says nothing about the changes in the situation and cannot see every factor. Remember MJ and I were told "three to five years" and had thirteen.

HOW YOU LIVE FOR HOWEVER LONG YOU HAVE
REMAINING AT THE MOMENT IS MORE IMPORTANT THAN
ALL THAT HAS COME BEFORE—THIS IS HOW YOU WILL
BE REMEMBERED.

Doctor number four was diametrically opposed to number three. "You're relatively young and in otherwise good health, if we can remove the new tumor while preserving an acceptable quality of life, why not? And let's change from Temodar to Avastin. Just this week it's been approved for your situation."

It was this doctor that we followed. He was quite candid in explaining the procedure and the risks, but much of it was in terminology that shot past with hardly time to ask for clarifications. But with some visual aids I learned he would be doing a rather different procedure. Where the first surgeon removed a golf ball-sized tumor plus about 1/16" of brain, this next operation would take a marginally smaller tumor and the entire lower lobe in which it was imbedded.

The only way of evaluating this fire-hose of information and opinion was to reduce the jargon to options: #3 said he wouldn't perform second surgery; it would only reduce the quality of my time remaining without extending my time significantly. #4 said yes to the second operation because the tumor was in an operable position and unlikely to cause quality of life issues. I got through the first operation rather easily so a second operation seems a good choice.

What's important to note here is that with two diametrically opposed opinions, the decision is mine, not theirs.

> LISTEN TO YOURSELF,
>
> AND THINK HOW IT WOULD BE RECEIVED.

But, as an engineer, I'm not able to evaluate their professional opinions or skills, I have to leave out the emotion and reduce the situation to one of two probabilities. If I let emotions in, I'll be over their waterfall of panic and confusion.

But part of that non-emotional evaluation was to notice that doctor #3 was young, and #4 was nearing retirement. Yet their roles seemed reversed in that the younger doctor would, or so one might think, be the more optimistic physician. The logical question, then, is why would that be? A look at the background of each provided some insights. #4 had been teaching this procedure for years and, as such, had to constantly be in touch with the prevailing wisdom and the results of the procedure. Doctor #3 may well have had his opinion fixated on a few cases that went less than well.

The one thing I learned to ask after the tidal wave of jargon had passed was simple: "If I was your brother, what would you advise me to do?" And as he answered I looked straight into his eyes. If they looked at the floor I was not too sure they believed their own words.

All of these doctors are, I'm sure, very good at what they do. That it's open to a difference of opinion is, I suspect, why it is called a "practice." Keep that in mind when you listen to their words.

Tool #9 – Watching Your Words

Now that you've gotten the diagnosis and the friends and neighbors have learned of it, you are likely to be confronted with words of solace that don't quite sooth the soul. This is the subject that, at first infuriated me, and then became a source of calm, good words poorly stated.

In the time between that night of the red lights and now, I have received a lot of well-intentioned statements of sympathy that have not done much to cheer me up. In those weeks I have gone from being annoyed with some of the statements, angered by others, and incredulous at the insensitivity of some. Fortunately I have found a way around them that leaves everyone unscathed.

I want to relate to them, though, as a way to illustrate the journey, so here comes the bruising, and again, I apologize. Your intentions are appreciated, they truly are, but the effect is not what you intend. If you hear yourself in these little stories, perhaps you'll moderate what you say. As you read the next parts, however, be prepared for a totally different solution to the problem.

SORROW SHARED IS HALVED, JOY SHARED IS DOUBLED.

"You'll be in our prayers" is commonly said. But is it being heard the way it is intended? If the patient is of your religion, perhaps or not. Regardless of the speaker's intention, it carries an unintended message of "You are doomed and only the intercession of a God can help." Such slim odds are not quite a message of cheer.

If the listener is an agnostic or atheist it might be taken as condescending, as in, "You're about to find out that I was right... God will (I hope) forgive your sins." Is that what you, the speaker, intended to say?

If the listener is of another religion, it might even be an insult.

So how do you, the patient, reply? Several options come to mind; it depends on the depth of your convictions. You could get into a philosophical debate on the subject of religion, but given the obvious depth of their convictions, the intent of the statement, and your own health, a simple "Thank you" is sufficient, and then leave it at that. It is best to move on to the next-step issues.

Of course if you, the patient, are confronted by an increasing number of offers of prayer and if it disturbs you as much as it did me, you might have to confront the speaker. Try "I know you mean that with the best of intentions, but I'm finding the idea that only a miracle can help is a bit depressing. If it helps you to pray, please do, but could you instead just wish me the best?"

THERE ARE THOSE WHO WANT ETERNAL LIFE,
BUT CAN'T FIGURE OUT WHAT TO DO ON A RAINY DAY.
— MAGNUS WENNERHOLM

"It'll be okay." This is second on my list of what not to say. The generic insistence is made all the more difficult in that it often comes right in the middle of my trying to explain the situation.

I come from a scientific/engineering background that relies on evidence not hope; logic not speculation. And even if I did not have that as a basis, I can't help but think any recipient of the statement sees that it also carries a subtext of doom; that if we only wish hard enough, that if we all clap our hands, the poison that Tinker Bell swallowed will magically go away. Again, it is not only a denial of the facts; it is a refusal to listen, or to look for a practical approach. Here's a third recitation.

"Aunt Martha went through chemotherapy and is now miraculously cured." That's nice for her, but the assumption is loud: "You've got cancer." When I first started hearing this, I didn't have a diagnosis beyond "It's a mass that we need to remove." Stories that go beyond the current diagnosis are hardly what I want to hear, even if it is couched in positive terms.

One person told me that a relative had a similar situation and it turned out to be a totally benign growth that was nothing more hazardous than a high-level sliver in her thumb. No message of doom there, but it was still not quite as good as looking at the facts.

> BETTER TO SAY NOTHING AND BE THOUGHT A FOOL,
> THAN TO OPEN YOUR MOUTH AND REMOVE ALL DOUBT.
>
> — MARK TWAIN

There's no end to the **faux pas** that will come your way. A friend just called to ask how I was. I mentioned that I was starting chemotherapy next week and his immediate response was "You're going to be sicker than hell!" Fortunately I was able to counter that with newer information that today's therapies do not include the horrors of previous years. Regardless of the state of technology, though, his observation was not helpful.

Oddly enough, one of the most insensitive statements came from the first neurologist. Based on an out-of-place scribble on the EEG and a blur on a low-resolution MRI, he adopted a dour expression and started speaking of brain surgery that could impair motor functions, affect the ability to speak, impede balance when walking, and cause slow mental acuity. It left the general impression that I ran the risk of becoming a drooling subject of pity left to sit in my diaper over in the corner.

My fears were magnified when he asked if I traveled overseas recently. I had not, but was curious as to why he'd ask. "Some foods carry parasites that can lodge in the brain." Shades of Stephen King! For a split second the scene in the movie "Alien" where the monster bursts out of its victim's chest played before me!

Others have done this gracefully, you can too. The clincher was his telling me that without treatment, I had a median of three months to live; with treatment, perhaps twelve. You'll recall that those numbers were later corroborated by other physicians, but this doctor's timing left something to be desired.

In all fairness, I brought this response on myself by asking worst-case scenario questions. But then, I'm new to this; he's not. My questions should have been deflected inside by an emphatic "Don't go there, you'll just scare yourself. We can discuss that if, and when, the evidence indicates it. All we know now is that something is not correct and we need another test to define the problem."

At the top of the list of unsettling statements is one I received after my previous wife died: with a hand on my shoulder and loving voice I was told that **"God must have wanted her more than you."** I was outraged at the idea that if I loved her a bit more she'd still be here. I know he thought he was saying something comforting, but it has been many years since I heard that, and it still stings to recall it.

During a visit to the hospital for a blood-draw, the phlebotomist asked about my health. I told her about my brain cancer. She responded with a story in detail about how her husband had this and how they were in denial right up to his death. She spoke of the anguish at such length I found my sympathies were all for her. When we were done I gave her a hug and wished her well.

Now, here's the really ironic part. Even after writing this I find that I have to really jerk my own leash when speaking with another person with cancer!

I'm prone to take off with my own tales of stupid statements instead of listening to them. If the conversation comes around to this, fine. But don't assume they're ready to kick that ball around. And even the pro's such as the chaplain or the speaker at the Cancer Help Group can blow it.

The meaning of all this, you may wonder. You, the patient, will have to learn to be just that, patient with people who unwittingly dump a lot of crap on you. With a little practice, though you can turn it to fertilizer.

That realization eventually, and thankfully, morphed into my rule of looking only at the next step.

The lesson here is simple:

1. Think before you speak.

2. Determine if what you're about to say is of benefit to the patient or just you.

3. If you can't remember to ask what the next step is, say nothing beyond "How are you?"

THE BEST QUESTION TO ASK A CANCER PATIENT?
WHAT'S THE NEXT STEP?

Tool #10 – Making Fertilizer

Of course, if I'm on the receiving end of one of these or other gaffs, what can I do if my rehearsed responses just don't work, or I am worn out by this seemingly endless verbal duel? Short of making a sign saying "Ask me what's next" and sticking it onto my forehead, is there much I can do, as the patient?

I have found a philosophy that takes practice, but has become easier than it sounds. Also, a success or two showed an immediate benefit.

It goes like this:

If someone gives me a gift and I refuse it,

who then owns the gift?

Obviously, it's the giver.

Hence, if someone says something that hurts or seems callous and I refuse it, then the feelings and pain that go with the gift are never received.

The adviser? Buddha some 2,500 years ago. Reinventing the wheel for all those centuries, aren't we?

Holding that tool close, I found that writing this started in anger and morphed into a learning experience. How to get to that state requires some understanding. First, try to understand why good people can say bad things. The answer is, I think, they're scared. Saying nothing leaves a void: the news is a shock. Perhaps they're even thinking "It actually could happen to me!"

> IF SOMEONE GIVES ME A GIFT AND I REFUSE IT,
> WHO THEN OWNS THE GIFT?
> — SIDDHARTHA GUATAMA, 500 BCE

All of this is a motivation to say something, if only to show they understand a bit about it, even if they don't.

Once I absorbed this idea, I found that the flame of anger diminished and that knowledge, in turn, allowed me to refuse the "gift." I was able to remove a rock from my back pack as I continued on my journey up the mountain.

At the buffet

To achieve this state, listen to your own response. I cataloged my responses over time and found there were six levels:

A.   Quiet pain – the remark hurt, but in a way I couldn't define. It was just mixed in with the shock of the situation and it couldn't be seen as a separate issue.

B.   Anger – "Knuckle-head!" Now it's an item akin to getting a parking ticket; just one more irritant.

C.   The rejoinder – "Gee, thanks, that was really helpful." I spent time thinking up snappy comebacks to dim-witted remarks.

D.   Polite but pointed – "Did you say that for me or for you?" Ouch! A couple of these, though, and you see that you have hurt someone that meant you well.

YOU'LL DO IT IMPERFECTLY. SO WILL THOSE YOU LOVE.
LEARN TO BE KIND TO BOTH YOURSELF AND TO THEM.

E.   Ignore it – this is much like the quiet pain. The sum of the hurts may be less, but the fact that this is from a friend makes it all the more difficult. What's the next step?

F.   The Gift Refused – Now I can have someone drop a bomb and simply say thank you. I take the part of the gift that I want and not accept the part that hurts. They don't know that I have done this and I'm warmed by their concern. We both win.

You could, of course, try to gently educate them in the art of saying what you need to hear. But that has a couple of drawbacks: first, they'll be stunned and hurt at their gaffe; second, you'll quickly be worn out by the constant repetition; and third, your friends will become nervous about what they say.

Your goal here is your own peaceful climb, not to educate the masses. With the knowledge of their intent, and a clear view of your own state, you can take what's offered. Think of it as a buffet; you don't have to eat it all.

But what if the person hearing these words of "help" is the spouse?

If the patient is really fortunate in having a supportive spouse, that person is also trying to climb the mountain. For instance, my wife and I almost invariably refer to us both when speaking of this situation, "Do we have radiation therapy today?"

The main difference is that I, the patient, will be excused if I get grouchy or need to take a nap; she might not. So my advice to the spouse is the same as to the patient: don't accept the gift.

More importantly, the advice to the well-intentioned speaker is the same as before, but even more so. Listen more than talk; don't be a cheerleader, be a friend; and finally, say nothing without first knowing who you are helping, the listener or yourself.

THE SECOND-BEST QUESTION TO ASK A CANCER PATIENT:
WHEN WILL YOU KNOW SOMETHING MORE?

Tool #11 – Saying the Right Thing

Having spoken of all the wrong things to say, what's right? Start by listening without a long face.

But what can you say? "What's the next step?" is an excellent inquiry. You've acknowledged the state of affairs and encouraged me to do something; that I'm not a passive victim and that I have got a plan.

"When will you know something more?" says that you're truly interested in my situation.

"Do you know what it is?" helps me define the issue, and helps us both understand the seriousness of the situation.

Yes, it is a serious issue, so a joke is inappropriate, unless I make it. And if I make it, it is to put us both at ease, so listen and laugh if you think it is a good one or groan if it is not.

Tool #12 – Work on the Positives

Similarly, it is amazingly helpful to watch fun movies. Dr. Allan J. Hamilton, a specialist in brain tumor surgery in his book on the same subject, The Scalpel and the Soul, makes a very interesting point.

It is an acknowledged fact that in Haiti, a believer in Voodoo can die from a curse! Their belief is so strong that they simply expire! He then asks the inverse, "Can your belief in health affect the cancer?" Can positive "vibes" help?

I'll dodge the question by simply asking, what's to be lost by assuming it to be true? With that in mind I'll do what I can to expel the depressing things in my life. I love movies so I'll watch adventures where the good guy wins, romantic comedies and farce. But I also enjoy enlightening and educational subjects even if they are tough. History and documentaries are favorites of mine; gratuitous violence is not.

Now, take this idea from another vantage point. If you go to a psychiatrist once a week, you'll spend a good deal of money to have them tell you that you are okay as you are, that you are a person of worth, that you have a right to be happy, or that your life is not hopeless.

After you invest in that hour you then expose yourself to countless billboards, magazine ads, and hours of TV advertising telling exactly the opposite! You are inadequate without their product; you won't get the girl on your own, you need this hair gel; you won't get the girl without hair; you look terrible if you're heavy, have the wrong hair color, and on and on.

The best thing you can do is to use the TV, quit letting it use you. Watch what makes you feel good, mute the advertising, watch romantic comedy movies only, or even unplug the darn thing if you must. But quit buying into the idea that you have to subject yourself to all the negative input.

An oddly helpful statement came from my brother-in-law. He'd emailed a link to a YouTube video that showed an amazing scene of four lions attacking a baby Cape Buffalo. They chased the youngster into the river where a crocodile grabbed the rear of the baby. The lions dragged the youngster out of the river away from the crocodile, and then the adult buffalo chased off the lions.

"What in the world was helpful in that?" you're saying right now. In his email, my brother-in-law appended a "How are you doing?" So I answered with all the scary news and quipped that I wasn't sure if that video was about the baby buffalo or me; we both had lions and crocodiles after us. He replied immediately pointing out that the little buffalo got away.

Now, that's helpful; concern not condescension, facts not wishful thinking, and parallels that encourage without being too closely parallel. I had a good laugh at his really fast response, too.

> TELEVISION IS VERY EDUCATIONAL,
> EVERY TIME IT COMES ON I GO READ A GOOD BOOK.
> — GROUCHO MARX

More to the point, though, if you want to help a friend in a similar situation, ask for the facts and offer assistance. The seizure precludes my driving a car, so if you're going to the store, call to see if I need a ride. Along the way we can discuss the next step.

The invisible poison

You have a support group, I hope, but repeating phrases such as "What would I do without you" may be heartfelt, but the focus, even if only tangentially is on the illness. This only reminds us of all the problems without an offering of any next-step answers. It decreases the sense of normalcy that is so vital to keeping an eye on what's the next step.

Of course you should thank the speaker frequently. But the best thank-you is to show how much he/she has helped just by leading a normal life. We all know the situation and may even be waiting for "What's next?" So tell them, thank them, and then show them how important they are by having a cheerful day (ignore this problem without pretending it doesn't exist). Yes, you may die from cancer, but because everyone will die from something does not make it a constant subject of discussion.

The positives backfire

The biopsy came back with the worst possible news. To put it simply, time is not infinite anymore. The first neurologist gave me a median of three months to live without treatment. The neurosurgeon made it plain in the simplest possible

words, it's a Glioblastoma multiforme Stage Four; he could remove it, and chemotherapy and radiation would extend my median to twelve months.

He then went to some effort to explain that there are dozens of treatments in trial. But, he adamantly explained, I should look at the cost; not the monetary cost as the trials are typically free to the volunteers, but the cost in quality of time and a possible diminution of total time. That is, of what use is a treatment that extends my life a few weeks if the price is to be in a clinic for several months?

He summarized it that "If a better treatment was out there, we would all be using it." However accurate that may have been, it said nothing to his arithmetic of time in a clinic vs. extension of life. That is a down-stream decision to be based on the facts at hand when the decision point arises.

What this surgeon didn't directly mention, but implied, is the potential of becoming involved in a desperate last-ditch quest. If you're old enough to remember the actor Steve McQueen, you might also remember that he died of cancer in Mexico chasing the magic bullet in the form of powdered peach pits. His last quasi-public statement was from behind a barely-open door in a down-scale motel. That's not how I want to remember him. He's the hero riding a motorcycle across beautiful grassy fields, being chased by WWII German soldiers in "The Great Escape."

I hope you don't want to be remembered as hiding behind a door. I certainly don't. But at the same time, I won't shut the door on a reasonable option.

Tool #13 – Simple Questions
for Simple Answers

Read that tool title again; it is not backwards. You'll find a lot of snake-oil sales-men. Unfortunately, you can only rely on regulations, integrity and good inten-tions just so far in this realm where a flood of hyperbole surfaces from the internet and even well-intentioned friends.

The tools for climbing the mountain will be helpful in this regard, but perhaps require more skill in using, especially when we all want the answer that will make all this go away.

Let's go through the list of actual assaults on my wallet and then see how the hype can be sorted from those worth investigating.

First, keep in mind that your emotions and desires are running at warp-speed and the hype-sters know it and will play to it. Your task is to keep those factors under control and think it through, ask some questions, and listen for the ring of truth. What answer would you like? It is out there. But is it plau-sible? All you need do now is to concentrate on the next step, all else is an un-changeable past.

Here it is again; don't let your emotions intrude upon the decisions. First, let's look at the worst on the list. It comes via the internet – where else? I was able to find many unscrupulous or perhaps just self-deluded "doctors" in Eastern Europe that offered a 100% guaranteed cure, their first step is to turn over the

number of your credit card. Of course, they offered a money-back guarantee! Who's going to collect it if they're wrong?

This sort of assault on your bank account is easily shot down with a simple observation, if they had a cure, why are they not selling their discovery to the highest pharmaceutical company, retiring wealthy, and enjoying the glory? Doing this would enrich them, if that was their goal, and save thousands of lives, if that was really their goal. Well-intentioned friends will likely commend websites with "This will amaze you!" and "Please, please read this!"

I got several of those messages and, given the situation, thought there was nothing lost in checking them out. One was a video of what looked like a legitimate TV show interview with an oncologist. He showed a before/after camera view from within the cancer patients lung stating that only four days had elapsed between the two shots and the cancer was gone. Amazing, I'll admit.

But I asked myself a few simple questions and thought through some of his statements. For instance, he stated that "cancer is a fungus." So here's the simple question: "The techniques for identifying a fungus are easy and well-known; if this were true, why has this taken so long to discover?" Next, he repeatedly stated "it's white, that means it's a fungus. Look at a mushroom, they're white!"

Again, let's apply a simple observation rather than acceptance. He's saying that all fungi are white. A walk in the forest will prove that wrong.

His treatment is to soak the tumor in sodium bicarbonate. Now, I'll agree that sometimes the best solution is the simple one, but that seems a bit too easy given the research done in countless laboratories in the quest for the perfect anti-

YOUR TIME IS ALL THAT COUNTS,
DON'T SPEND IT ON DEAD-END PURSUITS.

cancer agent. Surely those labs test the excised tumor for pH; if sodium bicarbonate would kill it, the labs would have found that out decades ago.

With my skepticism meter on HIGH, I did another simple check; an internet search of his name immediately revealed that he's been relieved of his medical license, convicted in a wrongful death suit in his home country and is being sought by the police in another for fraud!

Having set aside that savior, a friend recommended a book whose internet advertisement claimed the same astounding results.

The skeptical meter went up due to the delivery. It read like the script for a late-night infomercial while saying nothing. It had endorsements by several MD's, of course, but still, it didn't give a single clue as to the recommended treatment; diet, magic pill, or crystal spheres?

The advertisement gave the email address of one of the physicians so I wrote to her and within five minutes got a reply, not from the physician but from the author. The meter jumped up when I read that the physician "… had passed on my letter." It seemed unlikely that the physician had been able to read my letter, pass it on, and the author had responded in less than five minutes. More likely, my letter had gone straight to the author.

My meter was up another notch.

But the author did not answer my initial question; how could he when I was asking if the doctor still endorsed the author.

Meter up one more notch.

I wrote back chastising the author for the poor presentation and, in turn, received a pfd-type file of the entire book.

Meter down a couple of notches.

But a quick scan of the book revealed a lengthy endorsement of that previous physician with the sodium bicarbonate cure. Continuing my scan of the PDF showed that part of the cure included copious helpings of fatty, red meat, butter and whipping cream!

I'll dodge the cancer by dying of a cholesterol-induced stroke! That drove the meter off scale and I quit wasting any more time on this. It was, I'll admit, good for a laugh.

Now, the point is not that the only person to believe is your doctor. I got another book recommendation that says that all cancers, in fact all disease, is caused by processed sugar. I mentioned it to another friend and he enthusiastically endorsed the idea saying that the book is right, buy it.

All disease is caused by sugar? That's a real stretch but the book was cheap and I trust these friends. So I bought it thinking that the worst that could happen is I would spend under $10 and maybe lose a few pounds by cutting the sugar out of the diet. A bit of reading showed no sodium bicarbonate cures, just a healthy diet low on preservatives and processed sugars.

I move my meter down a notch because he is not asking me for more money.

> YOUR TIME IS ALL THAT COUNTS,
> DON'T SPEND IT ON DEAD-END PURSUITS.

In reading the book I found that the author is offering historical facts and citing events and sources that I can check.

Meter moved down another notch.

Not all of historical connections make sense though. He's saying that as sugar consumption has gone up, so has a long list of diseases.

This is called ergo Hoc, Prompter Hoc reasoning. It means after this, therefore because of this. I call it the virgin in the volcano logic where we toss some cute lady to her doom and get good crops next Spring.

Meter up. However, as I said, what's to lose by a healthier diet, so I'll continue reading.

The last "sure cure" I came across that needs a skeptical check is a report that advocates injecting the active ingredient of marijuana, THC, into the tumor site.

Perhaps the healthy cells "get the munchies" and wipe out the bad guys! This is one that I was tempted to just laugh at until I noticed the source. The Journal of the American Medical Association! In this case the vehicle reporting the study is not a late-night infomercial, but the most prestigious magazine in medicine.

Meter moved down several notches.

The bad news is that the report is about a study being done in Spain and so far has only tested two humans. So, while it might have some credibility, it is far too early to buy tickets to Madrid. Maybe someday.

The internet is a great tool for misleading you. But it can also be used to extract the realities from the rest of it. But for that to happen, you must set aside your wishes and desperate dreams. Does this make sense? Is this plausible? And remember, if it sounds too good to be true, it probably is.

At the other end of the spectrum, several years ago I participated with my previous wife in a study to determine if attitude affects the quality or duration of the patient's life. I don't know the outcome of the study and I really don't care. After all, what's to lose by assuming that a positive attitude helps?

An internet search will supply answers and supposed experts to relieve you of some cash to learn what the "doctors don't want you to know."

Tool #14 – Explaining "It"

During radiation therapy I spent a short period every day for six weeks in a waiting room. We became a "family" much as a group of soldiers under fire would. It was surprising to find that those with non-life-threatening cancers had little trouble in this arena; they were able to adjust to the situation, if not easily, at least in a fashion more akin to having been in a car accident. Friends simply asked, if anything was said, "How's it going?" For these patients it was more of a strictly internal acceptance issue.

For those of us with cancers that caused us to lose hair, and especially for those who had been told that it was a terminal situation, the reactions of friends were completely different. Some patients told me that their entire group of friends simply quit coming around. It was clear, I was told, that the news simply scared their friends; they didn't know what to say so they had taken the route of avoiding contact.

The casual acquaintance that might know you had a surgery asks "How are ya'?" The answer here is "Well, it's not so good. I just had brain surgery for a tumor that was successfully removed (positive spin), but the long-term prognosis is not good (truth). We're working on it though. (truth) How are you?" This lets them, and you, off the hook.

The neighbor/friend that knows I had the seizure and the subsequent surgery asks "Did you get the results of the biopsy?" This is a bit tougher. I started by taking them aside, sitting down and reciting a set-speech that begins with "First, listen to the sound of my voice; I'm not going to pieces so, as I explain this, understand that there is more to come." Then I would lay it out in a 1-2-3 factual way with an emphasis on the next step, and request that they not speculate. It would keep me from falling apart, and them from racing ahead with questions or being stuck in an "I don't know what to say" dilemma.

Then there is the family member/very close friend that knows some of it, but hasn't heard the latest news. Possible exchange:

Q. *"How are you feeling?"*

A. *(Open your arms and get a hug.)*

The constant repetition of the state of affairs became depressing and could have become a cause for people to avoid me. At least it seemed that way. However, it does not have to be the case! For me the key here was to share the news, first with my spouse/best friend, then with others. The more open I was, the more people gathered around.

After a week of seclusion with my wife and a lot of tears, I no longer avoided the question of "How did the surgery go?" We live next to a small, private airport and happened to arrive home from the surgery just as one of the neighbors landed with a new airplane. One of my very best friends, Gene, saw us pull up to the house and dashed over to tell us "Rob's arriving with the airplane!" We left the

> ### THERE ARE NO STUPID QUESTION,
> ### ONLY THOSE WHO CAN'T GIVE A SMART ANSWER.

car doors and trunk open and walked out to greet them and were fortunate that in the excitement and the oohs and aahs no one asked about my situation.

Gene walked back to the house with us and I had to simply blurt out "The doctor says that without treatment I have got three months, with treatment maybe twelve." My wife then invited him in for coffee and we spoke at length, all of us fighting the tears that still come even as I write this.

After listening for some time about how difficult it is to discuss this, he advised that "We need to rehearse our lines." I loved him for the "we" and the "our."

We talked of what to say and to whom. Over the course of a few days and several performances I have found that it became, if not easier, at least less emotional by dividing up my lines in several groups based upon the audience.

Rule One – "Oh what tangled webs we weave when we practice to deceive." It's not easy to keep the story straight even in the best of situations, so I have learned to be as truthful as I need to be, without being more truthful than is warranted.

The checkout clerk asks "How are you?" Even though it is pretty obvious they don't really want to know, this simple inquiry delivers a jolt (I was managing to ignore it until you asked!). The best thing to say? "Working on it." That's truthful, without too strongly reminding myself of the situation.

There are folks I have to call with the latest information. It is the same speech as for the neighbor/friend. The important part though, is that you should not wait for them to call you. You should call them so that you're prepared. Make

the call as soon as you're under control and know what you're going to say. Then do it when it is convenient for you both. If you can, get your friend and their spouse on the phone at the same time. Your condition is a burden for your friend as well, and he will not find digesting it is easy. You had a hard time with it, so will he. His spouse will be able to help him get his hands on all that you've said instead of him being burdened trying to explain it her.

There's another group of well-intentioned, but inexperienced people around the patient. They don't mention religion, magic bullets, or stories of cures; they just don't listen. In trying to explain what has happened, and how I'm feeling, I have sometimes been interrupted by their stories and comments to the extent that no information is passed and no feelings are calmed.

It makes me realize that this group—well-intentioned though they may be—have not taken the time to ask themselves why they are calling/visiting. Is it for themselves? To them I would advise that they ask their question, and then listen to the answer. Are they doing this for me? Then listen to what I'm saying. If they have another question, I'm open.

How do I handle them? I ask them to please just listen for a few minutes; it is the best gift they could give. If they still have questions when I have done my talking, then I'll do my best to answer.

I have had to listen to myself as well, though. I liken it to long-distance running; we've each got a limit and when we hit that wall we've got to stop. When that happens, I simply explain it by saying "Telling this is exhausting. Let's take a break." It seems to help both them and me by allowing them off the hook. I have

also found that suggesting that we go get a cup of coffee brings the relationship back to some semblance of normalcy before we break contact.

Still, why do the well-intentioned not listen?

Psychotherapist I am not, but it seems that the behavior is an indicator of their fears; they want everything to be okay; they don't know what to say, but they are more afraid of being distant.

To this group I would say only that you will be a help to your friend in need and to yourself by carefully thinking about what you want to accomplish before you pick up the phone.

After a few months of this fencing I learned to, as The Buddha said, refuse the gift and found the easiest tool of all, humor.

When asked "How are you feeling?" I now respond with open arms, a silly smile, and "Come find out!" It always gets a warm hug from the person asking, it breaks the tension with everyone and even causes a line of ladies to form.

Tool #15 – Recognizing the Part
That Sneaks up on You

Halfway through the chemotherapy and radiation therapy, I had an insight. I'm fighting the disease, but I'm also being assaulted in two other ways: first the C/R therapy makes me physically weaker by about 1% per day. But in doing so I'm finding it easy to feel weaker than I physically am.

I started using a cane just for stability to walk; now I'm leaning on it even if I don't need to. It has become a crutch in both senses of the word. I have been playing a role, watching to see how other people react. It's insidious! From that day forward I vowed to see the cane for what it is; a temporary assist. Of course I'll take advantage of the temporary Handicapped parking when I feel the need, but I stopped playing the role of the person who is permanently afflicted. This cane is a medical tool just as is, say, a cast on a broken arm.

The second assault comes from the most well-meaning people: they assume I am handicapped to the extent of my display with the cane. Their voices become sad when asking something as innocuous as "How are you?" It feeds that mental state I have addressed above and then lays a pressure back on me to be as weak as they expect … I don't want to disappoint them!

In short, there is a feedback loop here. I'm down, you're sympathetic, I respond by being more down, you respond by anticipating every need, I don't want to disappoint you so I'm further down … and on and on.

The other side of this coin is that I don't want to pretend that I feel fine when I don't. Pretending that all is just dandy could cause me to actually drive myself to really needing to be leaning on the cane. The middle road is best: use the cane, but don't let it use you.

Tool #16 – Keeping Control of It

For any of the people to whom you've explained anything, go on to ask that you would prefer that they not divulge those details for three reasons.

One, if someone asks them "How's Bob?" give your friend some "lines." The best one might be similar to the "casual acquaintance" approach, that is, "Well, it's not so good. He just had a brain surgery for a tumor that was successfully removed (positive spin) but the long-term prognosis is not good (truth). They're working on it though (truth). How are you?" And, once again, this lets both your good friend and the listener off the hook.

The second reason for this approach is that it minimizes the inevitable blur that occurs after you tell Joe, who tells Fred, who tells Mary. In the first weeks, those details will be changing daily so, in addition to the "blur", there's a lack of completeness even if the story is repeated perfectly.

Are you religious? Use your minister, rabbi, priest or whatever the title; it's their job. But again, I would suggest that the "Good friend/family" approach is best.

And while you're at it, include your spouse in these discussions if they're up to it. Remember that they are affected even more than you. Right now you might be saying "How's that possible?" The answer is simple, your problems, should the worst happen, will be over but your loved one will go on.

Surprisingly, I found that my emotional energy level has a limit that

extends to even the non-health issue. I had a falling out with a good friend last year prior to this issue. I was asked "How's so-and-so doing?" and inasmuch as I was in my honesty mode I explained at great length how the falling out occurred and everything that had transpired since then. Afterwards I was exhausted.

In sharing with my wife we came to the conclusion that all I should have said was "no change" and left it at that. I have only just so much energy and that lengthy explanation wasn't necessary

The bottom line on all this is that I'm learning to accurately divulge what I need to without doing a data-dump on those who can't take it, and that includes me.

By making it easier on them,
you make it easier on you.

THE SOLUTION!

How to share the latest information about myself with everyone was a problem. My friends truly want to know and I knew I would get asked the same questions or be confronted by friends who did not know what to ask. So I beat them to it by writing a health newsletter and sending it out to a mailing list of "surgery friends" after each change or check-up.

This openness was paid back by friends vying to take me to treatments. I, in turn, invited them in to see the radiation machine. Nick took some wonderful photos and I wrote an explanation of how it works. Later, we did the same thing with the MRI.

When I saw a friend, the conversation was now about how they have to have an MRI and they're glad to know what to expect. What a switch!

You can see a few of the newsletters at

http://whatsthenextstep-swansborobob.blogspot.com/

DEVOTE YOUR THOUGHTS TO WHAT'S LEFT,

NOT WHAT'S LOST.

Tool #17 – Getting the Affairs in Order

Nor am I a lawyer so I won't give legal advice except to say you should see one while you're capable. You do a huge disservice to your family if you leave your estate in limbo. You may be thinking that the spouse will inherit everything so there's no need to worry about it, everything will be straight-forward. This is not the case.

When my previous wife was near the end we made out a will. And even though her sister is a lawyer, we waited literally to the day before she died to do it. That's not a pleasant occupation at any time, and a gigantic misuse of that last day, week, or month.

Additionally, the will had many mistakes that might have been caught had it been taken care of earlier. It was an unneeded stress to work these out in the days after she passed.

Getting all this in order in my case included finding my Navy Discharge papers, the title to a tiny property I inherited, and going through the safety-deposit box and, most importantly, my deciding who of my friends and family should get what. That last item is not a burden I want to leave to my dear wife.

And while I'm at it, I should go out to the workshop and figure out what to do with unfinished projects. Put all the parts in one group and sell it, even if it is only for pennies on the dollar. At the minimum it keeps you active. After all, that it is unfinished is most likely because you lost interest; so with that attitude, simply clean out the garage.

One of those things my wife said she'd like to do is to go out to the workshop and help me clean out. It is a way of sharing time and getting closer to the hobbies I loved.

So, I guess I should do the same thing with my clothes closet. I haven't worn that pair of pants since they shrank around the waist. So I'll donate them and save my spouse a burden. I don't think of this as erasing myself from her life. If I want to work on it or wear it, I'll keep it.

A stickier problem comes about when you, the patient, start designating which friends get which items. Keep in mind that, if you're lucky, your best friend is your spouse. Don't give away anything without asking two questions: one, will the item be needed as a financial support for your spouse? Two, does it have a sentimental value to your spouse? You "earned" these items together; they should be disposed of in the same way.

My wife tells me that she's in a quandary; on the one hand she wants to continue to run her small company so as to keep a sense of normal life for us both. On the other, she feels that she might be wasting the time we have, but a big part of her wants to concentrate on the here and now.

We're fortunate in that we can take a few weeks off from work, but even so some balance has to be struck. Just as I shouldn't ignore the need to clean the shop in the best times, I can't ignore the big picture of making a living.

Completely unforeseen was that having cleaned up all these areas, we both feel great . . . Why didn't we do that a long time ago?

HOPE SUSTAINS LIFE,

MISPLACED HOPE SUSTAINS WASTEFUL PURSUITS.

Tool #18 – So How Do You Keep
Everyone Informed?

That first, high-definition MRI came with the news of the tumor and I was not looking forward to repeating the story twenty times. We had been invited to a dinner party to be held the night I got home, and I decided that the best way of dealing with this was simply and quietly, to announce it one time and to everyone at the same time.

That way they all have all the facts, they don't have to ask a question (somebody else already did) and I don't have to start from zero again and again. It was simply put, with no tears or speculation and a minimum of words. I explained what we knew, which wasn't much, what we did not know, and most importantly, what would be the next step. (There are those three words again.) When someone went on a tangent, I simply pulled it back to the next step. Very quickly everyone became interested in the realities instead of speculating. That had the benefit of putting the party back on track and, within just a few minutes, all was normal.

That technique of telling everyone simultaneously was extended to an email/newsletter in which I apologized for not making it one-on-one and then explaining my reasons. It gave me time to compose an accurate statement and, as it turned out, allowed them time to read it, absorb it, and compose a response. Everyone agreed that it was a good technique and the universal response of "how can I help" was amazing.

During the radiation therapy stage I invited one or two friends at time

to see the machine. Using Nick's photos, I released as a tongue-in-cheek "news bulletin" describing everything. The positive response has left me in tears. I never knew I had that many really true friends.

You'll remember Voltaire with his principle of Enlightened Self-Interest; here it is again. They get to hear what they can't ask and I get paid by their interest in me.

Much is said about keeping a positive attitude; little is said as to just how to go about it. Are there tools for that part of the journey? That gets an emphatic YES!

My son recently wrote asking to hear the stories of my life. He said that he needed to know his ancestry so as to help define himself; that without that knowledge he'd be nothing but a punctuation mark in the book we call the family history.

So I have responded by telling him of the time I asked my grandmother the same question and how amazed I was to hear that the first of us in America was smuggled in, hiding in a barrel because he was a dwarf. This was at a time when any handicap was an automatic bar to entry.

Later I told my son about my grandfather, a man who pulled himself out of alcoholism to become the relative I loved the most. Flowery prose was not needed, just the then-there-was-the-time stories; the sort that we've all related over a beer at lunch. I related the a story of the summer my grandfather and I spent three days digging with pickaxes to recover a huge underground gas tank and how, later that year, I got a check for $20 as my part of the profits.

Little stories, fun or sad stories … they all are wanted by someone, if not now, then later.

But for you, the patient, writing them will be a release from the intrusion of cancer; you'll be able to ignore it, to relax, to laugh, to realize what's important.

> JUST AS A WELL-SPENT DAY BRINGS A HAPPY SLEEP,
> SO A WELL-EMPLOYED LIFE BRINGS A HAPPY DEATH.
> — LEONARDO DA VINCI

Tool #19 – How do You Say "No" to Well-intentioned Visitors?

First, recognize that the patient (you?) is the primary concern. My friend Gene laughingly suggested "Work it for all it's worth!" The point of his statement was not that the disease should be a tool for selfish behavior, but that it must be recognized by everyone that the patient may have simply run out of emotional or physical "gas." As I went through radiation to the brain, I found that I was down in energy about 1% every day.

The reality of it is that I have friends that could love me to death and I have to sometimes simply take a nap. Consider how they would feel if they knew they were imposing; it is better to say something. So what to say?

"I would love to see you, but I really need to take a nap" will work every time. It is as simple as that. Your friends will understand, and if they don't, well, it is their problem.

Tool #20 – Who's in Charge Here?

My mantra for many years has been "Who's in charge here, emotions or logic?" Now that I see that I have been climbing a mountain and the top is within sight, I'm facing the end in a square-on fashion, instead of stumbling along. I am finding that repeating the question "What's the next step?" is essential if I'm to make the most of my time remaining.

Now, I have to emphasize that "facing the end" does not mean I have a fixed expiration date. There's that "median" again!

Consider this: life is a terminal illness and has no survivors. The median is not a deadline. I could be hit by a bus tomorrow. What it means is that I have been given a gift. I have been reminded of my mortality in such a fashion as to allow me to clean things up and say I love you.

I don't intend to sound too Pollyannaish. Instead I'm pointing out that although the silver lining in this cloud is the flash caused by the bolt of lighting that nailed me, I will be better served in putting it to use by keeping a cool head.

This might be the toughest of all the things you do. Simply put, don't panic. Given the state of affairs, this is likely to be very difficult.

Go ahead and cry; go out into the forest and yell if you must. But when you've exhausted that reservoir, look at what remains and use it. Don't speculate, don't chase the magic bullet, and don't waste too much time on tears. Keep in mind what's been said about that slippery term "median" and review what's left instead of what's lost.

If you're religious, embrace it. There's a better life awaiting you and you have time to affirm those beliefs assuring your place.

If you're not religious, that is to say you believe that life just ends, don't worry, there is nothing going to happen.

Either way, it is not too bad. The hard part is not death, they are the steps you take between now and arriving at the top of the mountain. This is the journey over which you have control, if you'll just take it.

Crossing the glacier

Extending the metaphor of climbing a mountain, there is also crossing the glacier.

As I go up this mountain I have learned that a spouse/friend is vital to making the trip a bit easier. It is impossible for anyone to maintain a positive outlook at all times. Indeed, if someone were to do so, they would be a candidate for the couch. But to be positive in this situation is, on the one hand difficult, and on the other hand necessary if I'm to avoid wasting what time is left.

This mountain is not a simple pile of rocks, it includes slippery glaciers, potential avalanches, and yawning crevasses. On any climb, there will be missteps on the small, round stone or my foot will slip sideways. Those are the times when I see what faces me and feel depressed. But like a mountain climber, I cannot announce my single foot-shift to the support crew; to do so is to place too much burden on them. It also makes me focus on the slips instead of the view.

At the same time, I cannot remain silent when the missteps are with both feet and I am scrambling to simply stay upright; this is where my spouse/friend grabs an elbow until I get my feet back under me. To stay silent at this point is to let myself slide down the glacier into depression where tears are the only focus.

The Grim Reaper will come to take me to the top if I don't do the climb myself, so I have a choice: I can climb the mountain enjoying the view; or I can slide down the glacier into the crevasse, remaining there until he finds me.

Tool #21 – A Friend Has Abandoned You in a Time of Need. Now What?

This could be one of the tougher issues to deal with. That old adage that a friend in need is a friend indeed is not a fully definitive idea. For instance, you need help moving furniture, but your buddy has a bad back and can't be there for you; is he any less of a friend?

So it is with emotional issues; some folks just never learned how to deal with them. The only thing for you, the patient, to do is forgive them for their inability.

Again, don't waste time on what's lost; spend your energies on what's left.

YOUR TIME MAY BE SHORT,

DON'T WASTE TOO MUCH OF IT CRYING.

Tool #22 – Troubles Shared Are Halved

My wife's family lives in Sweden and we have decided to visit them. Then I got to dwelling on the mechanics of saying goodbye for the last time; to go home to die. It was really depressing, I was even afraid to share it with her. But I did and her response was simply to remind me again what the term "median" means.

The important point here is not the meaning of "median"; we've been through that. There's another adage that says "Sorrow shared is halved; joy shared is doubled." In this case, sharing my fears caused them to evaporate.

The upside of this is that we are closer now than we've ever been because we've learned that when one of us is weak, the other can help. Try it in the following parts.

The day-to-day

In a recent movie titled "Making Waves", the female lead tells a guy-friend that now that her boyfriend has moved out she misses seeing his used towel on the bathroom floor. "Well" he says, "that's what bathroom floors are for!" With this knowledge, and lot of hilarity to come, the guy and girl get together. They realize that it is the tiny things that make a relationship; that it is easy to love one another when on that big vacation, but it is the tough times, and how we handle the trivial, that are the measure of the relationship.

With that knowledge it would seem obvious that a re-surmising of what's important is in order. So, ask yourself this: In the big picture of the situation, is this or that really important?

This applies to the seemingly callous remarks made by a visitor as well as our own short temper. "No, it's not fair; no, you don't deserve this." But more to the point, that's irrelevant in that you can't change it; to shout "Unfair!" is to look backwards; you're wasting time and energy on un-fun pursuits. Indeed, there is no fair or unfair in this: there just "is."

The other side of that coin, though, goes back to the principle of enlightened self-interest. Do what's best for all concerned and everyone is better off, including you.

Sliding off the glacier and into the crevasse

When I joined the Navy, the first thing done was everyone's hair was cut as a way of leveling the social distinctions. We all were nervous about how we would look, but as we realized we all looked the same, the fears wore off and we laughed about it.

Some years ago, with rapidly thinning hair, I cut it all off and polished the ol' dome as an impulsive experiment in being "hip". I found that was more trouble than it was worth to keep it polished. I let it grow back.

While in chemo and radiation, I grew tired of looking at the hair clogging the shower drain and finding it on the pillow. So I went to the barber and had my hair cut to about 1/16" inch. Having been in this state twice before I thought it would be an easy transition.

That length didn't work too well, though. Imagine a very stiff toothbrush being moved forwards and backwards on the pillow; it drags the pillow with it creating a very uncomfortable night.

Later, we were driving to our home some three hours away and stopped for coffee in a shopping center. On impulse, I bought an electric razor and was able to plug it into the car's power so, as we continued our journey with my wife at the wheel, I proceeded to polish the noggin, telling my wife, "Hey, if Patrick Stewart can make this look good I'll give it a shot."

I was laughing at the guy in the car behind who must have been thinking "Can't that bozo find an ear for his cell phone?" Then I heard a cheerful beep-beep and looked to the right to see a stunningly good-looking brunette in a hot

red sports car giving me a three-finger sign with perfectly manicured nails while she mouthed "I love it". My wife laughed too as the brunette shot around us to swing into our lane and those lovely nails popped out through the sunroof with that same sign of approval. My day was "made."

But the approval wore off as I continued my journey up the mountain. Even in the best of circumstances I have to sit down, yet I can't be the cheerful hiker enjoying the view all the time. However, even when sitting, the journey continues.

Later I shaved my head because I was looking a bit mangy. But, unlike those previous forays into smoothness, it felt as if it had become a sign hanging around my neck saying in large print "He's sick." I had been losing it on top for years, but that was just the process of growing older; shaving the head has become a glaring neon sign that screams that I'm unlikely to continue that path or that I'm now on a path where I can see the end. Then I felt that should not have done it. I walk past a mirror and am reminded: I feel the breeze on the back of my neck; I scratch an itch … and I'm reminded. There's no respite. I'm not ignoring the cancer; I'm not pretending that it's not there. But I would like to not be constantly reminded of it.

Oddly enough, letting it grow back was worse. The radiation stunted the growth in large areas leaving me looking like a map of the Greek Isles. So I shaved and hoped for another cute brunette to drive by.

For sanity we need rhythm and predictability. Hence the changes and progress we, as a species, so admire are largely the purview of the young. Now

I understand the loss my previous wife felt when she lost her hair to continued medication. When she was in the midst of that transition I thought it not that tragic; that I would have been losing it for years; that our society puts too much focus on hair.

Now I understand that it is not the loss that weighs us down, it is the sign we pick up that screams "Cancer Victim!" It is something that each cancer patient must deal with; just know that It is only hair, not you.

With that absorbed I went back to polishing the noggin. And then the actuality of it appeared: It really is just hair and a rather popular style at that.

When you bought that new car all of sudden you noticed them everywhere. So goes it with this new display of non-hair. Today I actively counted men with totally smooth heads. I found five just at lunch and the oldest was in his early forties!

Now, before you grab the razor, here's the bottom line: It is a nuisance to maintain. Two days without shaving and you "stick" to the pillow. If you choose to be smooth, buy a floating-head electric razor that will conform to the hardness and roundness of the skull and plan on doing it nightly while watching a movie. And look for that cute brunette in the red sports car.

All this is fine if you're a man. Mary Jane, however, bought a nice wig. It wasn't a perfect solution but it worked. She then made lemonade from lemons by buying a collection of dramatic hats. No turban for her! And it was great fun to

have the maitre d' light up when such a stylish lady showed up. It reminded me of the wonderful hats worn by Audrey Hepburn in "My Fair Lady".

I enjoyed it enormously and I think everyone else, including MJ, had great fun. It became an excuse to do something I suspect she always wanted to do.

Perhaps you've wanted to be a redhead? Do it. Remember that this is your permission to have some fun—no one will say "no."

Tool #23 – The Upside of It All . . .
There Actually Is One

Earlier I mentioned my previous wife, MJ, and that she had been told that she had three, perhaps five years to live when she was a mere forty-two years old. That gave us the impetus to "just do it." And we did. She decided that she was not going to live long enough to collect the savings from her 401K, social security and all the rest. I, on the other hand, would inherit/collect it all. Therefore, I did not need to worry about savings too much and neither did she. The upshot is that we lived for thirteen years as if she had three to five.

We did a refinance on the house and took out $30,000 in equity to pay for new carpets, drapes and other home improvements. And then, having withdrawn the money, we got out a couple packages of Post-Its, and on each page wrote out our really-want items, including the drapes and carpeting, with a rough idea of price.

Next, we arranged them in columns on the kitchen table that totaled $30,000. If we really want that $10,000 item, we'll have to remove items totaling $10,000. After an hour of this we found that carpeting and drapes were off the list. An extended tour of England, along with several lesser items was, literally, high on our list. Neither of us ever regretted it.

Now my current wife, Li, and I have decided to visit her family in Sweden. That insidious curve with its "median" shows survivors out to eight years;

perhaps I'll be one. But whether I make it that far or not, we're moving in the right direction.

It took three tries though; we bought trip insurance so we were able to change tickets, and a good thing. At the finish of chemo and radiation the tumor had grown back.

Rather than panic we simply asked what the next step is. There it is. No panic, no crying, no howl of "unfair"; It just "is".

This was a test of my ability to keep the emotions under control. Who is in charge here, the emotions or the intellect?

But how do you plan the trip? Again, think it through to arrive at a best-for-all decision. I have a choice: Start a new chemotherapy or undergo another surgery. The surgery will remove this tumor, the chemo has a 25% chance of being effective. The choice is easy; do the surgery, then the chemo.

When to leave for Sweden was decided by logic, not impulse. The chemo should show a result after two or three bi-weekly treatments and has an effect that should allow me to skip a treatment or two. So, do the surgery, then the chemo; if the chemo is working, take the trip. The chemo will be waiting. If the chemo is not working, then take the trip and enjoy myself while I can.

This is an example of using one of those decision-making tools. Think through the facts with the emotion stripped out, then go on to the next step.

The spouse's journey

Along the climb you will have noticed, if you're fortunate, that a spouse or close friend has aided your journey. They cannot, of course, go with you to the top. But how they respond to your journey can make the climb very hard, or much easier on themselves and on you.

Again, you have the control and, hard as it may seem to believe, you have the easier burden; you can show a courageous face to the world and people will admire you for it, but if the spouse does the same they may be thought of as uncaring or callous.

So, oddly enough, the patient has more control here. The spouse is a tool that can help the journey and, like any tool, it must not be abused; but to be useful, it must be used. If they are worn out, give them a rest; if you are worn out, employ their support. If both of you are feeling exhausted, rest together perhaps not saying a word. But the key is honesty and recognizing that in your climb of the mountain, they, too, are under a heavy load. When my MJ finally reached the top of the mountain I saw that we had each been through the Kübler-Ross stages in our own way.

She walked into our house, sat down and had a stroke. I called the doctor and was told that he could do nothing other than give her a bed in the hospital. MJ was able to speak and stressed upon me "Truth". I relayed what the doctor had said and she smiled. She then asked "How long?" and I said "Two days, maybe a week". I asked if she needed anything, she said "No, I'm at peace".

For the next three days we had a never-ending stream of friends and family visiting, with MJ never being alone. When she died at home I was angry at the doctor for not doing anything. But within a minute I realized that he would have if he could. I then accepted the inevitability of death and realized that her fears as she approached the event had been avoided by her constant focus on the next step. She had, in her graceful walk up the mountain, given me a gift.

For several weeks afterward I went to bed thinking that this is the longest I have ever gone without seeing her...and that tomorrow night will be a new record. But I was able to think back to her graceful steps and I realized that in so doing she'd relieved me of a load of my own.

But then, I had to walk back down the mountain. The journey had it's version of the Kubler-Ross model. I was distracted by the unfairness that a person who was loved by everyone she knew should be taken at the age of 55.

I was angry; I wanted to die in her stead. These ideas almost consumed me until I got back down off the mountain. Today I see these emotions as signposts indicating a natural path that we will all find on the mountain.

YOU CAN'T MAKE A DEAL TO GET YOUR LOVED ONE BACK.
MOVE ALONG THE SPIRAL OF LIFE.

The bottom line in a bumper sticker

There's a bumper sticker that says "He who dies with the most toys wins". I never believed it then, and I don't believe it now. The true measure of anyone's life is this: "He who dies with the shortest list of things he wishes he'd done is the winner."

So now, I have that gift that few receive; I have the time to tell those I love how I feel; to mend fences; to reduce, as was so beautifully described in a 2009 movie of the same title, "The Bucket List". In it, two friends work to reduce that list of things they wish they had done. If you've not seen the movie, find it and enjoy with a dear friend.

I would propose a new bumper sticker: "He who dies with the shortest bucket list, wins."

The essence of this was well expressed some five hundred years ago by Leonardo de Vinci when he said, "Just as a well-spent day brings a happy sleep, so a well-employed life brings a happy death." It is that sense of trying for comfort in my last days, of having done it well, of having left a gift of grace in the face of the inevitable that motivates me to write this. I wish to leave behind a gift to family and friends: a guide book on climbing the mountain.

At the minimum, I try to always keep in mind that the most important thing is the next step; even if it is only to say "I love you".

Realizing that there is no escape from the climb up the mountain is the first step in learning to enjoy the view ahead. I am fortunate to have many, especially the meandering waters of Rock Creek.

Then again, the doctor made a guess, not an expiration date. I'm thinking of the future because there is one no matter how.

MAKE A "BUCKET LIST" OF THINGS TO DO,
THEN DO THEM AS BEST YOU CAN.

Epilogue – Using the Tools

Here's a real world experience. I had lunch with a friend I have not seen in several weeks. His first comment was that he thought I was a pretty strong person for my taking it all in stride. He went on to tell me that he had been to a dinner party with a brain surgeon. Ben mentioned me to this doctor and was told, "Your friend (me) has maybe three months to live."

I stumbled over that bit of loose rock and grabbed the tool box rather than crash over the precipice!

Tool one: There's that time frame being referred to as if it were a label on a milk carton, dispose of after three months! I'm way beyond that time and feeling fine so I can dispose of the number instead!

Tool two: Eating at the buffet. Take only what I want. And what I choose to hear is that Ben takes my situation even more seriously than before; now he's gotten corroboration from an independent expert. What I won't take is the opinion of an expert who's making a diagnosis and prediction without seeing the patient or even the records.

The doctor in question showed himself to be rather insulated in giving an opinion with so little data. How many people might he have panicked with such idle comments? So combating the expert took another tool: the realization that the doctor does not always keep his oath to "Do no harm", even if he's correct in his words.

Was my friend Ben saying this for his benefit or mine? Perhaps it was for

WHEN SOMEONE SAYS SOMETHING THAT HURTS,
YOU MIGHT BE LISTENING TO YOUR OWN PHILOSOPHIES
OR PRE-CONCEIVED IDEAS.
TRY LISTENING TO THEIR HEART.

the both of us. He has a family member undergoing a serious medical issue right now so it might well have been a chance for him to stand away from that trouble for a brief moment while he considered my situation. His comment regarding my attitude was to say that he's using me as a guide in his own climb.

So, here I sit on the trail having stumbled on my climb. It has given me the time to consider the view though. I see a friend that has shown he cares about me; he has taken the time to learn a bit from an expert. He sees me as a strong person that he admires. That's a pretty nice view.

Another time I just came from the doctor; I have a third tumor. It's bean-sized and located outside the area of brain that was removed during my second surgery ten months ago. Evidently the individual tumor cells have scattered to other locations. We feared this might happen and had rehearsed what we would do or say if the news was bad.

We had, of course, picked up another tool: Set the emotions aside and think. So with emotions calmed down, we discussed the options with the doctor, found the best path. I'll be adding a new medication to the brew. It's called CCNU; I take it orally once per six weeks, then take an anti-nausea pill for three days or so. While medication works its way through me, I'll also be treated by a new machine called the Cyber-Knife. I'm told that this is a computer controlled, tightly focused beam of radiation that can incinerate the tumor without cutting the scalp.

After a couple of minutes of feeling somehow betrayed I again reached into my box of tools and brought out my favorite one. You remember "what's

next"? Li and I got our emotions under control, looked at the schedule and went to a different part of the hospital for a scheduled blood draw. That took care of that next step; the next step was to then call some good friends and meet for dinner under an early evening sun at a sidewalk restaurant. Now we're home, Li is working on her business and I'm writing this.

Now the next step is to write a newsletter to my Surgery Friends mailing list. I'll just send these paragraphs and later I'll write a detailed report on how the Cyber-Knife works. But at the moment, I'm keeping the emotions under control and just looking at "what's next".

Acknowledgements

I would like to thank fellow brain tumor patient, Victor Valdez, for arranging the manuscript in publishable form, coming up to Swansboro in the Sierra Foothills to work on the final draft and most of all for his moral support. Without his assistance, this book project wouldn't have been completed.

The Brain Tumor Support Group at Stanford University Medical Center has been a wonderful gathering of hikers on the BT journey. We were guided by Sharon Lamb and Joanie Taylor, retired registered nurses, who continue to care.

In our Swansboro community, the people have been extraordinarily helpful. We have developed many close relationships and consider them more than just friends. The gathering of locals at nearby Rock Creek Café on Wednesdays is truly a family night.

I benefitted from the professional care of the staff and physicians at Kaiser-Permanente topped off by their personal attention to patients such as myself. I extend my gratitude to the superlative Snowline Hospice, which continues to support me with end-of-life issues, as well as, moving *What's The Next Step* toward publication.

I would also like to thank those who found themselves on this journey especially for their openness to share their experiences. A handful had a chance to review advanced copies of *What's the Next Step?* Their comments and support of this project are greatly appreciated.

www.ingramcontent.com/pod-product-compliance
Lightning Source LLC
Chambersburg PA
CBHW020431290526
45785CB00002B/792